# Somatic Exercises for Weight Loss

## 30 Daily Practices for Physical & Emotional Well-being (Including Exercise, Flexibility, Strength & Balance)

### Helen Talbott

## Disclaimer

The information contained in this book is for educational purposes only and should not be construed as medical advice.

The author does not guarantee the accuracy or completeness of the information provided and disclaims any liability for any damages arising out of the use of the information contained herein.

Readers are advised to consult with a healthcare professional before beginning any new exercise program, especially if they have any pre-existing medical conditions.

It is important to note that individual results may vary, and the exercises presented in this book may not be suitable for everyone.

By using the information in this book, you acknowledge and agree to the terms of this disclaimer.

*"Weight loss is a journey, not a destination. Embrace the practice, not just the outcome, and you'll discover a world of well-being that extends far beyond the scale."*

# Table of contents

# Chapter 1

# Introduction

**Welcome to a journey of transformation!**

Have you ever felt trapped in a cycle of restrictive diets and frustrating exercise routines? Do you long for a deeper connection with your body and a sense of well-being that extends beyond the number on the scale? If so, then this book is for you.

This is an invitation to embark on a transformative journey through the practice of **somatic exercises**. Unlike traditional exercise, which often focuses solely on outward results, somatic practices offer a holistic approach to well-being. They guide you to connect with your body's inner wisdom, learn to listen to its signals, and move in ways that are both gentle and effective.

This book is your guide to unlocking your inner potential through the power of **30 daily somatic**

**practices**. We'll explore the **science behind somatic exercises and their unique benefits for weight loss, stress reduction, and overall well-being**. You'll learn about **warm-up techniques, essential exercises for different fitness levels, and how to build daily routines** that fit seamlessly into your life.

Whether you're a seasoned fitness enthusiast or just starting your journey towards a healthier lifestyle, somatic practices offer a path to lasting change. This book provides you with the tools and knowledge you need to move beyond quick fixes and discover a sustainable approach to well-being that nourishes your body, mind, and spirit.

**Are you ready to unlock your inner potential and step into a world of holistic well-being? Let's begin!**

# Welcome

I warmly welcome you to this exploration of **30 Daily Somatic Practices for Physical & Emotional Well-being**. Perhaps you've embarked on numerous fitness journeys, seeking weight loss or a stronger, healthier you. Maybe you've even felt frustrated by the limitations of traditional exercise routines.

Whatever your path, this book offers something different. It invites you to delve into the world of **somatic exercises**, a practice that transcends mere physical movement. Somatic practices bridge the gap between body and mind, nurturing both through gentle, mindful exercises.

Here, you'll discover more than just a collection of exercises. You'll embark on a journey of **self-discovery and empowerment**. We'll explore the **benefits of somatic practices** for weight loss, stress management, and overall well-being. You'll learn how to **listen to your body's unique signals**, fostering a deeper connection with yourself.

This book is your companion on this transformative journey. It provides **clear instructions, illustrations, and daily routines** tailored to different fitness levels. Whether you're a seasoned athlete or just starting, you'll find accessible practices to integrate into your life.

Get ready to **unleash your inner potential** and experience a holistic approach to well-being. Let's begin your journey towards a healthier, happier you!

# How to Use This Book

**Your Guide to Somatic Transformation**

This book isn't just a collection of exercises; it's an invitation to a transformative experience. So, grab your curiosity, a comfortable space, and get ready to embark on a journey of self-discovery through somatic practices. Here's how to unlock the full potential of this book:

**1. Approach with Openness:**

Leave behind preconceived notions of exercise and embrace the unique world of somatic practices. These exercises are more than just physical movements; they are conversations with your body, designed to cultivate awareness, not just physical results.

**2. Start With Your "Why":**

Before diving in, take a moment to reflect: what motivates you in this journey? Is it weight loss, stress reduction, or simply a desire to feel more connected to your body? Identifying your "why" will fuel your motivation and help you personalize your practice.

## 3. Explore the "Science":

Dedicate some time to understanding the **science behind somatic exercises**. Part 2 of the book delves into the benefits these practices offer, from weight management and stress reduction to improved flexibility and body awareness. Understanding the "why" behind the "how" can deepen your engagement and appreciation for the practice.

## 4. Warm Up and Stretch:

Every journey starts with a foundation, and in this case, it's your warm-up and stretching routine. Dedicate a few minutes before each practice to gently prepare your body for movement. Refer to the dedicated section on warm-up and stretching techniques to ensure you approach your exercises safely and effectively.

## 5. Choose Your Level:

This book offers a variety of exercises categorized by difficulty level (basic, intermediate, advanced). Start by exploring the **basic exercises** to establish a strong foundation. As your confidence and ability grow, gradually progress to the **intermediate and advanced sections**. Remember, consistency is key, so prioritize enjoying the movements at your current level rather than rushing ahead.

## 6. Build Your Daily Routines:

The magic lies in consistent practice. This book provides **30 daily routines**, each offering a combination of exercises tailored to different needs and time constraints. These routines are designed to be easily integrated into your daily life, whether you have 10 minutes or an hour to spare.

## 7. Make It Your Own:

This book provides a framework, but you are the artist! Don't be afraid to **personalize your practice**. Modify exercises to fit your body's unique needs and preferences. Listen to your body's signals, and take rest days when needed. The key is to create a sustainable practice that feels good for you, not a rigid routine that feels forced.

## 8. Beyond the Physical:

Remember, somatic practices extend beyond the physical. As you move, pay attention to your **thoughts, emotions, and sensations**. This awareness can lead to powerful insights about yourself and your relationship with your body.

## 9. Embrace Self-Compassion:

There will be days when motivation dips, or exercises feel challenging. Be kind to yourself! Embrace the journey and celebrate even small victories. Remember, progress, not perfection, is the goal.

## 10. Keep a Journal (Optional):

Consider keeping a journal to document your journey. Reflect on your experiences, note any insights or challenges, and track your progress. This can be a valuable tool to stay motivated and celebrate your achievements.

This book is your companion on your path to a healthier, happier you. Embrace the exploration, listen to your body, and discover the transformative power of somatic practices. Remember, the journey itself is just as important as the destination, so enjoy the process of uncovering your full potential.

# Why Use This Book

**Unlocking Your Inner Potential Through Somatic Exercises**

Have you ever felt like your fitness journey has hit a plateau? Perhaps you've cycled through countless diets and exercise programs, yet haven't achieved the desired results or felt truly connected to your body. If this resonates, then this book offers a unique and transformative approach: **somatic exercises**.

Here's why **"30 Daily Practices for Physical & Emotional Well-being"** can be your guide to a healthier and happier you:

**1. Go Beyond the Scale:**

This book offers more than just weight loss strategies. Somatic exercises are not about chasing numbers on the scale, but about **cultivating a holistic sense of well-being**. By focusing on mindfulness, body awareness, and gentle movement, you'll build a healthier relationship with your body and experience lasting improvements in your overall health and well-being.

## 2. Unlock Your Inner Potential:

Somatic exercises go beyond the physical, unlocking a deeper connection between your mind and body. By tuning into your body's signals and moving with intention, you'll **discover hidden strengths and capabilities**, empowering you to reach your full potential and move through life with greater confidence.

## 3. Reduce Stress and Enhance Mood:

Stress is a major contributor to health problems and decreased well-being. Somatic practices, with their emphasis on mindfulness and gentle movement, are **powerful tools for stress reduction and mood improvement**. By calming your nervous system and fostering relaxation, you'll experience reduced stress, increased emotional resilience, and a renewed sense of calm.

**4. Build Sustainable Habits:**

Unlike restrictive diets and intense exercise routines, somatic practices offer a **sustainable and enjoyable approach** to well-being. By creating personalized routines that fit your lifestyle and preferences, you'll be empowered to **build lasting habits** that contribute to your long-term health and happiness.

**5. No Gym Required:**

This book offers a variety of exercises that can be done **anywhere, anytime**, without requiring a gym membership or expensive equipment. This makes it an accessible option for everyone, regardless of budget or limitations.

**6. Discover a Supportive Community:**

This book is your starting point, but you're not alone on this journey. We've included resources and information for further exploration, allowing you to **connect with a supportive community** of individuals interested in somatic practices and well-being.

This book is not a quick fix; it's an invitation to invest in your long-term physical and emotional well-being. By embracing the power of somatic practices, you'll embark on a transformative journey towards a healthier, happier, and more empowered you.

**Chapter 2**

# Understanding Somatic Exercises

## What are Somatic Exercises

Somatic exercises, unlike their more conventional counterparts, offer a refreshingly unique approach to movement and well-being. Stepping beyond the realm of simply burning calories or building muscle, they delve into the intricate tapestry of **mind-body connection**. But what exactly defines this unique practice? Let's embark on a journey to understand the essence of somatic exercises and explore the potential they hold for transforming your life.

**From the Greek Roots to Modern Practice:**

The term "somatic" originates from the Greek word "soma," meaning "body." So, in essence, **somatic exercises are practices that integrate the body and mind in a coordinated and**

**mindful manner**. These exercises go beyond just moving the body; they encourage you to **tune into your internal sensations**, fostering a deeper understanding of how your body moves, feels, and responds to different stimuli.

**Mindfulness at the Forefront:**

A cornerstone of somatic exercises is the **practice of mindfulness**. Unlike traditional workouts that focus solely on achieving a specific goal or performing a movement perfectly, somatic exercises emphasize **being present in the moment** and **paying attention to the subtle signals your body sends**. This heightened awareness allows you to identify areas of tension, observe your breathing patterns, and ultimately, move with a **greater sense of purpose and control**.

**Moving with Intention, Not Force:**

Gone are the days of pushing your body to its limits through repetitive motions. Somatic exercises **reject the notion of "no pain, no**

**gain"**. Instead, they encourage **gentle and intentional movement**, emphasizing **quality over quantity**. This shift in focus allows you to explore the full range of motion within your body without exceeding your limits or causing discomfort.

**A Conversation with Your Body:**

Imagine viewing your body not as a machine to be pushed and pulled, but as a **conversational partner**. Somatic exercises encourage you to **listen to your body's unique language** and respond accordingly. By paying attention to internal cues like fatigue, tightness, or discomfort, you can **modify exercises** and tailor your practice to suit your individual needs and limitations.

**More Than Just Physical Movement:**

The benefits of somatic exercises extend far beyond the physical realm. By focusing on **mind-body integration** and cultivating **self-awareness**, these practices can lead to significant improvements in your **emotional and mental well-being**. They can:

- **Reduce stress and anxiety** by calming the nervous system and promoting relaxation.
- **Enhance self-compassion** by fostering a kinder and more accepting relationship with your body.
- **Improve sleep quality** by promoting relaxation and reducing tension.
- **Boost mood and energy levels** by encouraging mindful movement and fostering a sense of accomplishment.

**Unveiling the Potential:**

Somatic exercises offer a path to **cultivating a deeper understanding of your body, mind, and emotions**. They empower you to move with intention, listen to your body's wisdom, and ultimately, **unlock your inner potential** for a healthier, happier, and more fulfilling life. It's an invitation to embark on a transformative journey of self-discovery, one gentle movement and mindful breath at a time.Benefits of Somatic Exercises

In today's world, the pursuit of well-being often leads us down a path of rigorous exercise routines or restrictive diets. While these approaches may yield results, they often miss a crucial element – the **mind-body connection**. Somatic exercises, with their unique blend of gentle movement and mindfulness, offer a refreshing and **holistic approach** to well-being, unlocking a spectrum of benefits that extend far beyond weight loss.

## 1. Cultivating Mind-Body Awareness:

Somatic exercises go beyond simply moving your body. They encourage you to **tune into your internal signals**, fostering a deeper understanding of how your body moves, feels, and responds to different stimuli. This heightened **mind-body awareness** allows you to identify areas of tension, observe your breathing patterns, and ultimately, move with a **greater sense of purpose and control**. Imagine gaining a deeper understanding of your body's language, learning to interpret its cues, and moving in ways that feel both **effective and sustainable**.

## 2. Weight Management Through Mindful Connection:

While somatic exercises may not be as calorie-intensive as other methods, they offer a more **sustainable and holistic approach** to weight management. By fostering a **mindful connection with food and hunger cues**, these practices can help you **curb emotional eating** and **make informed dietary choices**. You learn to listen to your body's signals, discerning between true hunger and emotional triggers. Additionally, the improved **body awareness** cultivated through somatic practices can support **intuitive movement**, encouraging you to engage in activities you genuinely enjoy, leading to a **more active and mindful lifestyle**.

## 3. A Haven for Stress Relief and Relaxation:

Chronic stress is a modern-day epidemic, impacting our physical and mental well-being. Somatic exercises offer a powerful antidote to this, acting as a **refuge for stress relief and relaxation**. The combination of **gentle movement and mindfulness** promotes the release of tension, **calms the nervous system**, and induces a state of **deep relaxation**. By focusing on the present moment and tuning into your body's sensations, you can **quiet the mind chatter** and find a sense of inner peace.

## 4. Cultivating Self-Compassion and Body Positivity:

Somatic exercises go beyond just achieving physical goals. They foster a **kinder and more accepting relationship with your body**. By focusing on mindful movement and exploring your body's limitations, you cultivate **self-compassion**. You learn to appreciate your body for its unique capabilities and move with greater confidence and acceptance. This shift in perspective can significantly improve your **body image and self-esteem**, allowing you to connect with your body in a positive and empowering way.

## 5. A Holistic Approach to Physical Well-being:

The benefits of somatic exercises extend beyond the mind and emotions. Gentle movements inherent in these practices can **improve flexibility, balance, and posture**, contributing to your physical well-being. By focusing on proper alignment and mindful movement, you can **reduce the risk of injuries**, improve your **range of motion**, and experience **greater ease and efficiency in everyday activities**.

### Embarking on a Transformative Journey:

Somatic exercises offer a **holistic approach to well-being**, encompassing your physical, mental, and emotional dimensions. By integrating gentle movement with mindfulness, they allow you to **uncover your inner potential, empower yourself to move with intention**, and ultimately, **cultivate a life filled with balance,**

**self-acceptance, and well-being**. It's an invitation to embark on a transformative journey of self-discovery, one gentle movement and mindful breath at a time.

**Chapter 3**

# Embracing Your Practice

# Warming Up & Stretching

## Warming Up Your Journey: The Importance of Pre-Exercise Preparation

Just like a car engine needs to warm up before hitting the highway, your body needs the same preparation before engaging in any physical activity, including somatic exercises. A proper **warm-up routine** is crucial for maximizing your performance, reducing the risk of injury, and ensuring a safe and enjoyable practice.

## Why Warm Up?

Here are some key benefits of dedicating a few minutes to a warm-up before your somatic practice:

- **Increased Blood Flow:** Warming up gradually increases your heart rate and blood flow, delivering vital oxygen and nutrients to your muscles, preparing them for movement. This improved circulation also helps **raise your body temperature**, making your muscles more pliable and reducing the risk of strains and tears.
- **Improved Flexibility:** A warm-up routine incorporating gentle stretches helps **lengthen and loosen your muscles**, increasing your range of motion and making it easier to perform exercises with proper form. This flexibility allows for smoother and more efficient movement, enhancing the effectiveness of your practice.
- **Enhanced Mental Preparation:** Taking a few minutes to warm up allows you to **transition smoothly from your daily routine to your exercise session**. This brief period of mindful movement helps **focus your attention, clear your mind,**

**and prepare mentally for the practice ahead**.

## How to Warm Up:

A proper warm-up should ideally last for **5-10 minutes** and consist of two main components: **light cardio and dynamic stretches**.

### 1. Light Cardio:

- **Start with 5-7 minutes of low-impact aerobic activity** that gradually increases your heart rate and blood flow. This could be brisk walking, jogging on the spot, jumping jacks (performed at a moderate pace), or arm circles.
- **Focus on maintaining a comfortable pace** and avoid pushing yourself too hard. The goal is to gently warm up your body, not to exert yourself.

### 2. Dynamic Stretches:

- **Dynamic stretches** involve controlled movements that mimic the movements you will be performing during your practice. They help prepare your muscles for specific activities and improve your range of motion.

- **Here are some basic examples:**
    - ○ **Arm circles:** Make large circles forward and backward with both arms for 15-20 seconds each way.
    - ○ **Torso twists:** Stand with your feet shoulder-width apart and gently twist your torso from side to side, focusing on keeping your hips facing forward. Hold for 10 seconds each side.
    - ○ **Leg swings:** Stand on one leg and swing the other leg forward and backward, keeping your core engaged and avoiding excessive hyperextension. Repeat for 10-15 seconds on each leg.

**Remember:**

- **Listen to your body:** Don't push yourself beyond your comfortable range of motion.

- **Breathe deeply:** Pay attention to your breath throughout the warm-up, focusing on slow and controlled inhales and exhales.
- **Transition smoothly:** After your warm-up, don't jump directly into your practice. Take a few moments to **transition mentally and physically** by focusing your breath and setting your intentions for the session.

By incorporating a simple yet effective warm-up routine into your somatic practice, you can **maximize your performance, reduce the risk of injury, and create a foundation for a safe and enjoyable experience.** Remember, taking care of your body allows you to move with greater ease and confidence, allowing you to fully embrace the transformative potential of somatic exercises.

**Chapter 4**

# Your Exercise Library

# Basic Exercises

Somatic exercises, unlike traditional workouts, prioritize **gentle movement, mindfulness, and body awareness**. They offer a safe and accessible approach to well-being, suitable for individuals of all fitness levels and abilities. This section delves into the **foundational exercises**, forming the building blocks for your somatic journey. Remember, these exercises are meant to be **exploratory and gentle**, focusing on **quality of movement over intensity**.

## 1. Mindful Breathing:

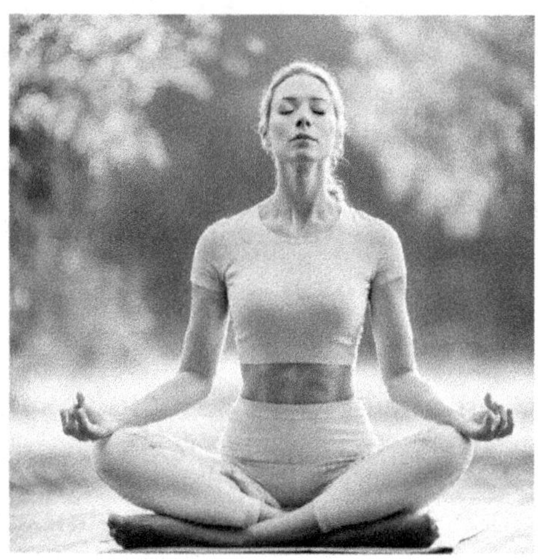

Somatic practices begin with the foundation of **mindful breathing**. Find a comfortable seated or standing position and gently close your eyes (if comfortable) or soften your gaze. Focus on your breath, observing the natural rise and fall of your chest and abdomen. Inhale slowly through your nose, feeling your belly expand. Exhale slowly through your mouth or nose, allowing your body to soften and release any tension.

Practice this for a few minutes, focusing solely on your breath and becoming aware of your body's sensations.

## 2. Body Scan:

This exercise fosters **awareness of your entire body**. Start by lying comfortably on your back with your eyes closed. Take a few deep breaths and begin to scan your body, starting from your toes and gradually moving upwards. Notice any sensations, such as tension, warmth, or tingling, in each body part without judgment. When you reach your head, take a few final breaths and gently roll onto your side to come out of the pose.

## 3. Pelvic Tilts:

Strengthen your core and improve pelvic awareness through this gentle exercise. Lie on your back with your knees bent and feet flat on the floor. Place your hands on your lower abdomen, just below your belly button. Gently tilt your pelvis down, pressing your lower back towards the floor. Engage your core muscles and tilt your pelvis upwards, arching your lower back slightly. Repeat this movement slowly and deliberately, focusing on the sensations in your abdominal and pelvic area.

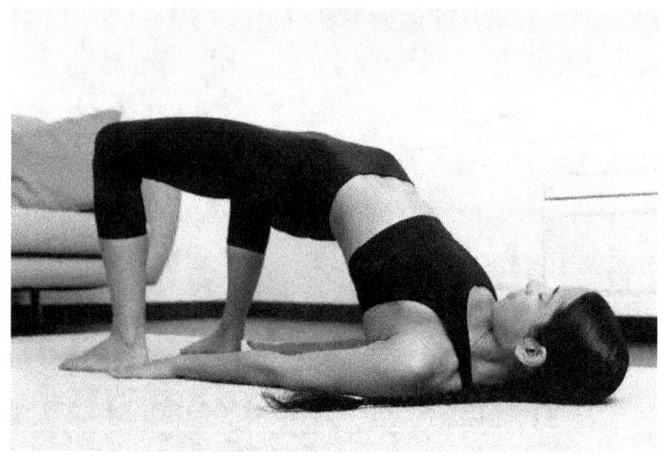

**4. Neck Rolls:**

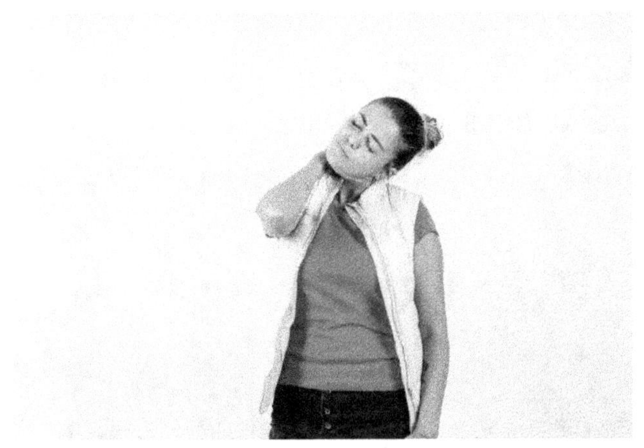

Improve your neck mobility and release tension with this exercise. Sit or stand tall and slowly roll your head in a circular motion, leading with your chin. Make 5-10 circles in each direction, keeping your movements gentle and avoiding any strain. You can also perform side-to-side neck rolls, tilting your ear towards your shoulder and holding for a few seconds before switching sides.

**5. Arm Circles:**

Enhance shoulder mobility and loosen up your upper body with this simple exercise. Stand tall with your arms extended out to your sides at shoulder height. Make small circles forward and backward with your arms, focusing on keeping your shoulders relaxed and your core engaged. Repeat for 10-15 circles in each direction.

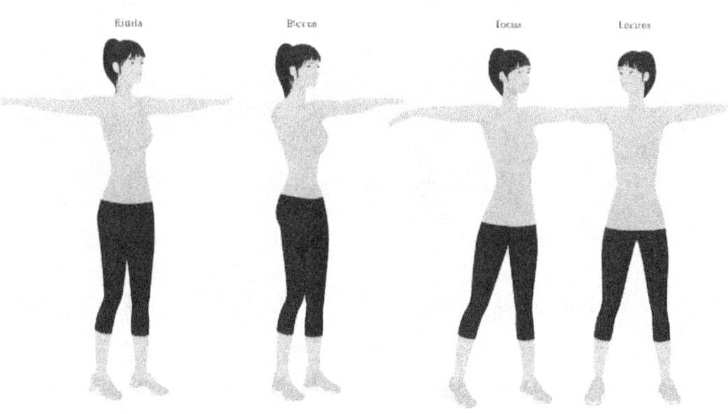

## 6. Gentle Spinal Twists:

Improve spinal flexibility and release tension in your back with this mindful practice. Sit on the floor with your legs crossed or extended in front of you. Gently twist your torso to one side, keeping your hips facing forward. Reach your arm out behind you and rest it on the floor or a chair for support. Look over your shoulder and hold for a few breaths. Inhale and return to center before repeating on the other side.

These are just a few **foundational somatic exercises**. Remember to **modify** them as needed to suit your comfort level and physical limitations. As you become familiar with these exercises, you can explore variations and gradually progress to more challenging movements, always prioritizing **mindful exploration and gentle engagement** over intensity.

By incorporating these basic exercises into your routine, you can begin to **cultivate body awareness, improve flexibility, and experience the transformative power of mindful movement**. Remember, **consistency is key**, so dedicate a few minutes each day to these exercises and witness the positive impact they have on your physical and emotional well-being.

# Embracing the Challenge: Exploring Intermediate Somatic Exercises

As you progress on your somatic journey, you may feel ready to explore more challenging exercises that build upon the foundational movements explored earlier. This section delves into **10 intermediate exercises** designed to gradually increase the intensity and complexity of your practice, while still prioritizing **mindful exploration and body awareness**.

**1. Downward-Facing Dog with Knee Lifts:**

**Description:** Start in a downward-facing dog position with your hands shoulder-width apart and your hips lifted towards the ceiling. Engage your core and alternate lifting one knee towards your chest, maintaining a flat back and keeping your gaze between your legs. Focus on controlled movements and feeling the connection between your breath and movement (5-10 repetitions each leg).

**Illustration:** (Image of a person in a downward-facing dog position, lifting one knee towards their chest)

## 2. Warrior II Flow:

**Description:** Start in a warrior II pose with your front knee bent and your back leg extended. Slowly shift your weight and raise your arms overhead, reaching towards the ceiling. Hold for a few breaths, then return to warrior II, and transition to the other side. Focus on maintaining a strong core and feeling the stretch in your hips and legs (3-5 repetitions each side).

**Illustration:** (Image of a person flowing between warrior II poses on each leg)

## 3. Side Plank with Hip Dips:

**Description:** Start in a side plank position with your elbow directly under your shoulder. Engage your core and lift your hips slightly, then gently dip your hips down towards the floor while maintaining a straight body line. Repeat for a few cycles, focusing on maintaining stability and feeling the engagement in your core and obliques (5-10 repetitions each side).

**Illustration:** (Image of a person performing a side plank with hip dips)

## 4. Cat-Cow with Arm Extensions:

**Description:** Start on your hands and knees with your wrists shoulder-width apart and knees hip-width apart. As you inhale, arch your back and look up into a cow pose. As you exhale, round your back and tuck your chin into a cat pose. Extend one arm forward and the opposite leg back as you exhale into the cat pose, and return to the starting position as you inhale. Repeat on the other side, focusing on coordinating your breath with your movement and feeling the stretch in your spine and shoulders (3-5 repetitions each side).

**Illustration:** (Image of a person performing a cat-cow pose with arm and leg extensions)

## 5. Bridge with Leg Extension:

**Description:** Lie on your back with your knees bent and feet flat on the floor. Lift your hips off the ground, engaging your core and glutes. Extend one leg straight up towards the ceiling, keeping your core engaged and your back in a straight line. Hold for a few breaths, then lower your leg and repeat on the other side (5-10 repetitions each leg).

**Illustration:** (Image of a person performing a bridge pose with one leg extended)

## 6. Mountain Pose with Arm Circles:

**Description:** Stand tall in mountain pose with your feet hip-width apart and your arms relaxed by your sides. Slowly make large arm circles forward for 10-15 repetitions, focusing on maintaining a long spine and feeling the stretch in your shoulders and upper back. Reverse the direction and repeat for another 10-15 circles.

**Illustration:** (Image of a person standing in mountain pose, performing arm circles)

## 7. Crescent Lunge with Twist:

**Description:** Start in a low lunge position with your front knee bent and your back leg extended. Reach your arms overhead and gently twist your torso towards the front leg, looking up towards your hand. Hold for a few breaths, then return to the starting position and repeat on the other side (3-5 repetitions each side).

**Illustration:** (Image of a person performing a crescent lunge with a twist)

## 8. Chair Pose with Arm Raises:

**Description:** Stand with your feet hip-width apart and squat down as if sitting in a chair, keeping your back straight and your core engaged. Extend your arms overhead and hold for a few breaths, focusing on feeling the engagement in your legs and core. Return to the starting position and repeat (5-10 repetitions).

**Illustration:** (Image of a person performing a chair pose with arms raised)

## 9. Warrior I with Side Bends:

**Description:** Stand in warrior I pose with your front knee bent and your back leg extended. Slowly reach your raised arm over your head and bend your torso towards your front leg, keeping your hips facing forward. Hold for a few breaths, then return to warrior I and repeat on the other side (3-5 repetitions each side).

**Illustration:** (Image of a person performing a warrior I pose with a side bend)

# Cultivating Mastery: Exploring Advanced Somatic Exercises

As your body awareness and confidence in movement flourish, you may desire more challenging exercises to further refine your practice. This section delves into **10 advanced exercises** designed to test your **balance, coordination, and strength**, while still emphasizing the core principles of **mindful exploration and body awareness**. Remember to approach these exercises with **caution**, modifying or omitting them if you experience any discomfort or lack the necessary preparation.

**1. Handstand with Wall Support:**

**Description:** Begin facing a wall with your arms shoulder-width apart and hands flat against the wall at shoulder height. Engage your core, kick your legs up one at a time, and walk your feet up the wall until your body forms a straight line. Hold for a few breaths, focusing on maintaining a strong core and keeping your gaze down towards the floor. Slowly walk your feet back down the wall to exit the pose.

**Illustration:** (Image of a person performing a handstand with wall support)

## 2. Single-Leg Balance with Arm Circles:

**Description:** Stand on one leg with your core engaged and your other leg lifted slightly off the ground. Extend your arms out to the sides and slowly make small circles forward and backward, focusing on maintaining your balance and feeling the connection between your breath and movement (10-15 circles each direction, repeat on other leg).

**Illustration:** (Image of a person standing on one leg with arms extended, performing arm circles)

## 3. Bird-Dog:

**Description:** Start on your hands and knees with your wrists shoulder-width apart and knees hip-width apart. Extend one arm forward and the opposite leg back, keeping your core engaged and your back in a straight line. Hold for a few breaths, then return to the starting position and repeat on the other side (3-5 repetitions each side).

**Illustration:** (Image of a person performing a bird-dog pose)

## 4. Side Plank with Leg Lifts:

**Description:** Start in a side plank position with your elbow directly under your shoulder. Engage your core and lift your top leg up towards the ceiling, maintaining a straight body line. Hold for a few breaths, then lower your leg and repeat for 5-10 repetitions. Switch sides and perform the same sequence on the other side.

**Illustration:** (Image of a person performing a side plank with leg lifts)

## 5. Downward-Facing Dog with Leg Lifts and Hip Circles:

**Description:** Start in a downward-facing dog position with your hands shoulder-width apart and your hips lifted towards the ceiling. Engage your core and alternate lifting one knee towards your chest, making small circles with your lifted knee as you bring it closer to your chest. Maintain a flat back and keep your gaze between your legs. Focus on controlled movements and feeling the connection between your breath, movement, and balance (5-10 repetitions each leg).

**Illustration:** (Image of a person in a downward-facing dog position, performing a hip circle with one lifted knee)

## 6. Warrior III with Arm Extension:

**Description:** Start in a warrior III pose with your back leg lifted and your arms extended at shoulder height. Extend one arm overhead and hold for a few breaths, maintaining your balance and focusing on feeling the engagement in your core and legs. Return to warrior III and repeat on the other side (3-5 repetitions each side).

**Illustration:** (Image of a person performing a warrior III pose with one arm extended overhead)

## 7. Chair Pose with Single-Leg Stand:

**Description:** Stand with your feet hip-width apart and squat down as if sitting in a chair, keeping your back straight and your core engaged. Slowly lift one leg off the ground and hold for a few breaths, ensuring your hips remain level and your core is engaged. Return to the chair pose and repeat on the other side (3-5 repetitions each side).

**Illustration:** (Image of a person performing a chair pose with one leg lifted)

## 8. Plank with Hip Dips and Arm Lifts:

**Description:** Start in a high plank position with your wrists shoulder-width apart and your body in a straight line. Engage your core and alternate lifting one arm off the ground, keeping your hips level and your body stable. As you lower the arm back to the ground, gently dip your hips down towards the floor while maintaining a straight body line. Repeat for 5-10 repetitions on each side, focusing on controlled movements and maintaining core engagement.

**Illustration:** (Image of a person performing a plank with hip dips and arm lifts)

## 9. Downward-Facing Dog with One-Leg Kick-Through:

**Description:** Start in a downward-facing dog position with your hands shoulder-width apart and your hips lifted towards the ceiling. Engage your core and quickly kick one leg up towards the ceiling, extending it straight

**Chapter 5**

# Crafting Your Personal Somatic Journey: Daily Routines for Well-being

Somatic exercises offer a unique approach to cultivating **well-being** by integrating gentle movement, mindfulness, and body awareness into your daily routine. Unlike traditional fitness routines, they prioritize **quality over quantity**, encouraging you to explore your body's capabilities with **curiosity and respect**. Here are some tips for incorporating somatic exercises into your daily life:

## 1. Start Small and Be Consistent:

Building a sustainable practice is key. Begin with **5-10 minutes** of somatic exercises a few times a week, gradually increasing the duration and frequency as you become more comfortable. Consistency is crucial, so find a time that works best for you and stick to it as much as possible.

## 2. Prioritize Mindful Breathing:

Every somatic practice begins with **mindful breathing**. Dedicate a few minutes each day to sit comfortably and focus on your breath, observing its natural rhythm without judgment. This simple act sets the tone for a mindful and present approach to your movement explorations.

## 3. Explore Foundational Exercises:

Start with **basic exercises** that focus on gentle stretches, body scans, and pelvic tilts. These exercises help you develop body awareness and prepare your body for more challenging movements. Refer to the previous sections on "Basic Exercises" and "Intermediate Exercises" for inspiration.

## 4. Listen to Your Body:

Somatic exercises are all about **tuning into your body's signals**. Don't push yourself beyond your comfortable range of motion or force yourself to perform exercises that create discomfort. Modify or omit any movements that feel uncomfortable, and adjust the intensity based on your individual needs.

## 5. Integrate Movement Throughout Your Day:

Beyond dedicated practice sessions, incorporate **mindful movement** throughout your day. Take the stairs instead of the elevator, stretch while waiting in line, or gently roll your shoulders while seated at your desk. These small movements can help you stay connected to your body and prevent stiffness.

## 6. Find Activities You Enjoy:

Somatic exercises shouldn't feel like a chore. Explore different types of movement, such as yoga, tai chi, or dance, and find activities that resonate with you and bring you joy. This will increase your likelihood of sticking to your practice in the long run.

## 7. Create a Supportive Environment:

Create a dedicated space for your practice, even if it's just a corner of your room. Use comfortable clothing that allows for free movement and consider playing calming music to set the mood. This dedicated environment can help you mentally shift into a space for mindful exploration.

**8. Connect with Others:**

Consider joining a somatic exercise class or online community to connect with others who share your interest. This can provide motivation, accountability, and a sense of community, enhancing your overall well-being journey.

**Remember, consistency, self-compassion, and a curious exploration of your body are the cornerstones of a successful somatic practice. Embrace the journey, and allow yourself to experience the transformative power of mindful movement on your physical and emotional well-being.**

# 30 Daily Somatic Practice Routines: Cultivating Well-being Through Mindful Movement

Somatic exercises offer a unique approach to **well-being** by integrating gentle movement, mindfulness, and body awareness into your daily life. This comprehensive guide presents **30 daily routines**, each outlining specific exercises and duration, to help you craft a personalized practice that aligns with your needs and preferences.

**Warm-Up (2-3 minutes):**

Start each routine with gentle movements to prepare your body and mind.

- **Mindful Breathing:** Focus on your breath for a few minutes, observing its natural rhythm without judgment.
- **Neck Rolls:** Slowly roll your head in circular motions, leading with your chin,

in both directions for 5-10 repetitions each.

- **Arm Circles:** Make small circles forward and backward with your arms, keeping your shoulders relaxed, for 10-15 repetitions each direction.

**Day 1-5: Foundational Focus (10-15 minutes):**

Lay the groundwork for your somatic journey by focusing on fundamental exercises that build body awareness and gentle mobility.

- **Body Scan:** Lie comfortably and scan your body from your toes to your head, noticing any sensations without judgment.
- **Pelvic Tilts:** Gently tilt your pelvis up and down, engaging your core muscles. Repeat 5-10 times.
- **Gentle Spinal Twists:** Sit or stand and twist your torso gently to one side, holding for a few breaths before repeating on the other side. Perform 3-5 repetitions each side.

- **Leg Swings:** Stand on one leg and gently swing the other leg forward and backward, maintaining core engagement. Repeat 10-15 times per leg.

**Day 6-10: Building Stability (15-20 minutes):**

Gradually increase the challenge by incorporating exercises that enhance core strength and stability.

- **Plank:** Start on your forearms with your body in a straight line, hold for 30 seconds to 1 minute.
- **Side Plank:** Hold a side plank position with your elbow directly under your shoulder, for 30 seconds to 1 minute per side.
- **Bridge:** Lie on your back with knees bent and feet flat, lift your hips off the ground and hold for 30 seconds to 1 minute.

**Day 11-15: Exploring Flexibility (15-20 minutes):**

Focus on gentle stretches to improve flexibility and range of motion.

- **Cat-Cow:** Move through cat and cow poses, coordinating your breath with your movement, for 5-10 repetitions.
- **Downward-Facing Dog with Knee Lifts:** Lift one knee towards your chest while maintaining a flat back in downward-facing dog. Repeat 5-10 times per leg.
- **Warrior II Flow:** Transition between warrior II poses on each leg, holding for a few breaths on each side. Repeat 3-5 times.

**Day 16-20: Strengthening the Core (15-20 minutes):**

Target your core muscles for improved stability and posture.

- **Bird-Dog:** Extend one arm and the opposite leg while keeping your core engaged and back in a straight line. Hold for a few breaths before repeating on the other side. Perform 3-5 repetitions per side.

- **Chair Pose:** Squat down as if sitting in a chair, keeping your back straight and core engaged, hold for 30 seconds to 1 minute.
- **Mountain Pose with Arm Raises:** Stand tall and raise your arms overhead, reaching towards the ceiling, hold for 30 seconds to 1 minute.

### Day 21-25: Balancing Act (15-20 minutes):

Challenge your balance and coordination with these exercises.

- **Tree Pose:** Stand on one leg with your other foot resting on your inner thigh or calf, hold for 30 seconds to 1 minute per side.
- **Single-Leg Balance with Arm Circles:** Stand on one leg and make small arm circles forward and backward, maintaining your balance, for 10-15

repetitions each direction, repeat on the other leg.

- **Warrior III:** Stand on one leg with your arms extended overhead, hold for 30 seconds to 1 minute per side.

**Day 26-30: Integrating Movement (15-20 minutes):**

Combine various exercises to create a more dynamic flow.

- **Mindful Walking:** Focus on your breath and body sensations as you walk, noticing the ground beneath your feet and the movement of your limbs.
- **Sun Salutations:** Flow through a series of sun salutations, coordinating your breath with your movement. Modify as needed.
- **Dance Exploration:** Move your body to music, focusing on expressing yourself

# Chapter 6

# Supporting Your Journey

# Cultivating a Healthy Plate: Basic Tips for Balanced Eating

Making healthy choices doesn't have to be complicated. By incorporating these fundamental principles into your daily routine, you can build a **nutritious and satisfying eating pattern** that supports your overall well-being.

**1. Embrace Variety:** Fill your plate with a **rainbow of colors** from different food groups. This ensures you're getting a diverse range of essential nutrients, vitamins, minerals, and antioxidants. Aim to include:

- **Fruits and Vegetables:** They provide essential vitamins, minerals, and fiber. Strive for at least 5 servings per day, with a focus on whole fruits and vegetables over processed options.

- **Whole Grains:** Choose whole grains like brown rice, quinoa, and whole-wheat bread over refined grains like white bread and white pasta. Whole grains are higher in fiber and complex carbohydrates, keeping you feeling fuller for longer.

- **Lean Protein:** Include protein sources like fish, poultry, beans, legumes, nuts, and seeds in your meals and snacks. They provide essential building blocks for your body and can help manage hunger.

- **Healthy Fats:** Include healthy fats like those found in avocados, olive oil, nuts, and seeds in moderation. These fats are essential for various bodily functions and can contribute to satiety.

**2. Prioritize Whole Foods:** Opt for **unprocessed or minimally processed foods** whenever possible. These foods retain more of their natural nutrients and fiber compared to their processed counterparts often loaded with added sugars, unhealthy fats, and sodium.

**3. Focus on Portion Control:** Be mindful of portion sizes, especially when consuming higher-calorie foods like nuts, seeds, and healthy fats. Use smaller plates and bowls, and avoid distractions while eating to facilitate mindful eating and prevent overconsumption.

**4. Limit Added Sugars:** Added sugars contribute to empty calories and can negatively impact health. Be mindful of added sugars in sugary drinks, processed foods, and even seemingly healthy options like yogurt and breakfast cereals.

**5. Stay Hydrated:** Water is essential for various bodily functions. Aim to drink plenty of water throughout the day, especially before, during, and after meals, and during physical activity.

**6. Cook More Often:** Cooking at home allows you to control the ingredients and portion sizes in your meals. This empowers you to make healthier choices and avoid the hidden sugars, fats, and sodium often found in restaurant and processed foods.

**7. Read Food Labels:** Develop the habit of reading food labels to understand the nutrient content of what you're consuming. Pay attention to serving sizes, calories, fat content, added sugars, and sodium.

**8. Listen to Your Body:** Eat intuitively by learning to recognize your body's hunger and fullness cues. Eat until you're comfortably satisfied and avoid overeating.

**9. Plan Your Meals:** Planning your meals and snacks in advance can help you make healthier choices throughout the day and avoid unhealthy impulse decisions.

**10. Enjoy the Process:** Make healthy eating enjoyable! Explore new recipes, experiment with different cuisines, and find healthy alternatives that satisfy your taste buds.

Remember, consistency is key. By gradually incorporating these tips into your daily routine, you can cultivate a healthy and sustainable eating pattern that nourishes your body and mind.

# Sample Workout Log Sheet

This template provides a basic framework for tracking your workouts. Customize it to fit your individual needs and preferences.

**Date:** ________

**Workout Focus:** (e.g., Strength Training, Cardio, Yoga) _________________________

**Warm-Up (5-10 minutes):**

- List specific warm-up exercises and duration (e.g., Light cardio - 5 minutes, Arm circles - 10 repetitions each direction)

**Main Workout:**

**Cool-Down (5-10 minutes):**

- List specific cool-down exercises and duration (e.g., Static stretches - 30 seconds hold per stretch)

**Additional Notes:**

- Include any additional observations or reflections about your workout (e.g., How you felt during the workout, areas for improvement, any modifications made)

**Tips:**

- Use a separate sheet for each workout or create a logbook for multiple sessions.
- Be specific about the exercises you perform, including sets, reps, and rest times.
- Track your progress over time to see how you're improving.
- Use this log to set goals and plan future workouts.

**Remember:** This is just a sample, and you can adjust it to fit your specific needs and preferences. The most important thing is to find a system that works for you and helps you stay motivated on your fitness journey.

# Conclusion

**Reflecting and Re-energizing: A Recap and Encouragement for Your Journey**

As you embark on your journey towards well-being, whether it's through somatic exercises, mindful eating, or any other path you choose, it's crucial to **pause, reflect, and acknowledge your progress**. This allows you to appreciate your efforts, identify areas for improvement, and most importantly, **rekindle your motivation** to continue your journey.

**Take a Moment to Recap:**

- **Review your goals:** Remind yourself of the initial inspirations and goals that set you on this path. Have they evolved? Are you still aligned with your initial vision?
- **Acknowledge your progress:** No matter how small, celebrate your achievements. Did you incorporate a new exercise into your routine? Did you make healthier

choices throughout the week? Appreciate these steps forward.

- **Identify challenges:** Be honest with yourself about any difficulties you encountered. Were there exercises that felt overwhelming? Did you struggle with certain aspects of healthy eating? Recognizing these challenges allows you to strategize solutions.

**Embrace Encouragement:**

- **Be kind to yourself:** Remember, progress isn't always linear. There will be bumps along the road, and that's okay. Embrace a compassionate approach towards yourself, accepting setbacks as opportunities to learn and grow.
- **Find your support system:** Surround yourself with positive and supportive individuals who believe in your journey and can offer encouragement when needed. This support can come from friends, family, online communities, or even a therapist or coach.

- **Reframe challenges:** Reframe challenges as opportunities for growth. Instead of focusing on the difficulty, view them as stepping stones on your path to self-improvement.
- **Celebrate small wins:** Celebrate even the seemingly insignificant victories. Every small step forward is a step towards your ultimate goals.
- **Focus on the journey, not just the destination:** Remember, the journey itself is an invaluable experience. Enjoy the process of learning, exploring, and discovering what works best for you.
- **Visualize your success:** Take time to visualize yourself achieving your goals. This mental exercise can boost your motivation and solidify your commitment to your journey.

By taking the time to **reflect, acknowledge your progress, and embrace encouragement**, you can **reignite your passion and stay motivated** as you continue your journey towards well-being. Remember, you are capable of achieving incredible things – keep going, keep growing, and keep thriving!

# Glossary of Somatic Terms:

**Basic:**

- **Body Awareness:** An awareness of your physical sensations and movements in the present moment.
- **Breathwork:** Focusing on and controlling your breath during movement or meditation.
- **Core:** The muscles around your abdomen, pelvis, and lower back that provide stability and support to your spine.
- **Mindfulness:** Paying attention to the present moment without judgment.
- **Modification:** Adapting an exercise to make it easier or more challenging, depending on your individual needs and abilities.
- **Posture:** The alignment of your body when standing, sitting, or lying down.
- **Range of Motion:** The extent to which your joints can move in a specific direction.

- **Relaxation:** Releasing tension and tightness in your muscles.

**Intermediate:**

- **Balance:** The ability to maintain your body in a controlled position.
- **Coordination:** The ability to use different parts of your body together smoothly and efficiently.
- **Flexibility:** The ability to move your joints through their full range of motion.
- **Proprioception:** Your body's awareness of its position in space and the movement of its joints.
- **Strength:** The ability of your muscles to exert force.

**Advanced:**

- **Flow:** Moving from one exercise to another smoothly and continuously.
- **Integration:** Combining different movement practices to create a holistic experience.

- **Proprioceptive Neuromuscular Facilitation (PNF):** A type of physical therapy technique that uses specific movements and pressures to improve proprioception and movement patterns.

**Additional Terms:**

- **Fascia:** A connective tissue that surrounds and supports your muscles, organs, and other tissues.
- **Somatic Exercises:** Gentle movements that focus on body awareness, mindfulness, and improving the connection between your mind and body.
- **Trigger Points:** Tight areas in your muscles that can cause pain and discomfort.

Remember, this glossary is not exhaustive, and there may be other terms you encounter as you delve deeper into somatic practices. Don't hesitate to research unfamiliar terms to gain a clearer understanding of the concepts involved.

# Bonus

https://go.screenpal.com/watch/cZef0rVKCxP

Video link for tutorials